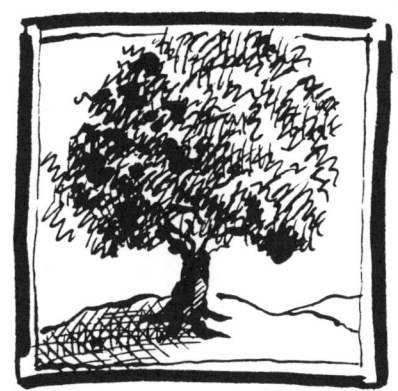

Wellness and Lifestyle Renewal

A Manual for Personal Change

Mark S. Rosenfeld, PhD, OTR

ΛΟΤΛ

The American Occupational Therapy Association, Inc.

Rockville, MD

Anne M. Rosenstein, Director of Publications

Edited by John Hutchins
Designed by Robert Sacheli
Art and Calligraphy by Elizabeth Wolf

Printed in the United States of America

ISBN 0-910317-92-5

This book is dedicated to my family with whom I share the complexity, promise, frustrations, and pleasures of discovering and creating our lifestyles together.

Special thanks to John Hutchins for his sensitive and creative editorial contributions.

Foreword and Instructions

A Preface for Therapists, Group Leaders, and Participants

Wellness and Lifestyle Renewal is written for "the worried well" and serves as a curriculum for therapists working in industrial and community-based health promotion programs. According to Barbara Rider, health promotion in occupational therapy is "the practice of informing, educating, facilitating behavioral change and using cultural support so people can assume responsibility for living a lifestyle that is centered on optimal well being" (Rider et al., 1989, p. 806). This book may be used either as a tool by occupational therapists or independently by nonprofessionals as a guide to practical personal change.

Unlike other wellness programs, which focus on single life issues such as fitness, stress reduction, smoking cessation, or time management (Dixon, 1988), *Wellness and Lifestyle Renewal* takes a comprehensive approach based upon the Model of Human Occupation. This model views occupation, the daily performance of purposeful activities, as the essence of human existence. According to Kielhofner, occupation "includes activities that are playful, restful, serious, and productive. These work, play, and daily activities are carried out by individuals in their own unique ways based on their beliefs and preferences, the kinds of experiences they have had, their environments, and the specific patterns of behaviors that they acquire over time" (Kielhofner, 1985, p. 12).

Modern life presents us with a great variety of life choices and responsibilities. Creating and maintaining a positive occupational status, therefore, cannot be taken for granted. Economic pressures, single-parenting, and high expectations for achievement and satisfaction all contribute to the challenge. Many people become overwhelmed with responsibilities and have little time for relaxation and fun. It is common for one to lose touch with specific activities and interests that were rich and absorbing in years gone by.

In general, it is hard to take real control over one's everyday choices and use of time. Given the complexity of life and the lack of simple formulas for self-fulfillment, many normal individuals need information, advice, and support in this regard. And yet, there are few resources available to help people look closely at the practical issues of life and to shape them in a positive way.

Occupational therapy has lifestyle theories, assessment tools, and change strategies to contribute to our efforts for fulfillment. Johnson (1986), a convincing proponent of occupational therapy involvement in the wellness movement, states that health and illness are fluctuating conditions strongly influenced by lifestyle factors. She stresses "the importance of viewing individuals as integrated organisms in which elements of mind, body, spirit, emotions, and environment are interrelated" (p. 757), which is a basic premise of occupational therapy. Therapists, Johnson insists, should move beyond symptomatic treatment to help people develop new visions of themselves and new contexts for living. My research with disaster victims has shown that lifestyle disruption can have a negative and disorganizing influence on people, but it can also stimulate a thoughtful process of positive change and personal growth (Rosenfeld, 1989). This workbook structures such a process, leading to lifestyle revitalization and change.

In *Wellness and Lifestyle Renewal*, concepts of lifestyle creation and management are introduced. Important quotations are highlighted so that they may be remembered, copied, and kept handy for inspiration. Exercises are offered at each step to promote a self-reflective and orderly method of lifestyle assessment and alteration. Information and insight gained from the exercises build toward concrete action plans in Chapter 13. Readers and participants can see their goals and priorities more clearly and embellish or rework the pattern of activities they live out each day.

The end result of *Wellness and Lifestyle Renewal* is a conscious, ongoing effort to:

- Know clearly what you want out of life;
- Pay attention to your most valued goals;
- Participate in activities you enjoy the most;
- Balance work, leisure, chores, and rest in a satisfying way;
- Manage your personal health, home, and finances effectively;
- Experience and deal with emotions well;
- Find intellectual stimulation and learn;
- Recognize and address your spiritual needs;
- Shape the places in which you work, recreate, and relax; and
- Create and maintain positive relationships.

This effort may seem like an overwhelming prospect. *Wellness and Lifestyle Renewal*, however, enables one to identify a target area of concern and take on manageable challenges one step at a time.

Wellness and Lifestyle Renewal may be undertaken in 5 to 10 sessions of individual consultation between an occupational therapist and a cognitively able client who is motivated to address lifestyle issues. Small group workshops offered through a community hospital health promotion program have been highly productive as well. Group members have generated new perspectives and initiated concrete changes within the context of four weekly sessions. Exercises may be completed in the office/conference room or as homework. It is best to proceed through the book and its topics in sequence. Some individuals, however, quickly recognize an area of concern after completing the first chapter and wish to move immediately to the relevant section. Such a jump is practical in working with a single client but may be too complicated for a group experience.

In a group, participants should discuss exercises in dyads and bring questions and conclusions back to the leader and the larger group. This approach establishes a strong and immediate source of support, advice, and information for each participant. Also, as Bronfenbrenner states, "Active engagement in, or even mere exposure to, what others are doing often inspires the person to undertake similar activities on her own" (1979, p. 6). The concrete, practical focus of the material encourages self-disclosure and feedback in a format that encourages rapid development of group cohesion.

A so-called "normal" population often demonstrates wonderful openness and creativity in completing the rather traditional occupational therapy assessments and approaches included in this workbook. It has been my experience in conducting *Wellness and Lifestyle Renewal* workshops that participants' views of their life issues evolve over 4 or 5 sessions. One woman, for example, began with only a vague sense of dissatisfaction, not with what she was doing, but with the way she experienced the events of daily life. Two sessions later, after completing an Activity Wheel schedule and a Role Checklist (see pp. 51 and 45), she cried bitterly as she recognized her pattern of intense self-deprivation; she worked hard professionally, but spared little time for relaxation, personal interests, or her preschool-age son. The woman resolved to shift her use of time so as to improve the balance among career, personal, and family activities.

A young man stated at the outset of a *Wellness and Lifestyle Renewal* workshop that he found it difficult to fulfill his graduate school assignments in the chaotic and noisy apartment that he shared with his roommates. He was prepared to move. In reviewing the chapter on social environments (see p. 57), the man recognized his long-standing pattern of shy sub-assertion and isolation. He had not connected with his roommates due to his reserve, nor had he attempted to negotiate with them about his concerns. The workshop group encouraged him to reformulate his renewal efforts toward acquiring assertiveness skills. He then used the Empty Chair exercise (see p. 89) to explore and address his conflicts about becoming more assertive.

Workshop participants' earliest statements often flag their most important process issues. A woman complained that she always asked "a million people's opinions" about life decisions, becoming confused and indecisive as a result. She retained little respect for her own judgment. The therapist and group agreed that she could fully explore her thoughts and feelings about subsequent decisions without interference. In the end, following self-reflective exercises, judgments, decisions, and discussions, the woman discovered that she had good common sense at her disposal.

These examples are offered to encourage therapists to actively guide and nurture the unfolding awareness of each participant. An ongoing flow of information, questions, and advice among participants and therapist is indispensable in this process. While the therapist acts as an expert consultant, workshop participants often have great strengths and resources to contribute as well. The following sequence of therapeutic steps that are typical of occupational therapy practice should be followed when conducting individual or group sessions of *Wellness and Lifestyle Renewal* (Rosenfeld, 1990, p. 55):

1. Address and examine functional history, current patterns, and future goals;

2. Reframe problems in a functional skill context;

3. Value and investigate the unique potentials, perspectives, and identity of the person;

4. Move from *reflecting* to *planning* to *doing* in a measured and productive sequence;

5. Offer expert consultation about occupational options, sequences, and performance;

6. Stress the person's responsibility for the decisions and actions that affect the quality of his/her life;

7. Use reality awareness as a template against which to view the person's decisions and actions;

8. Support growth through gradually developing skills, facing manageable risks, and accurately assessing productive efforts as well as end products; and

9. Foster the person's self-observing and problem-solving capacities so that occupational functioning will persist and improve beyond termination of therapy.

Variation in participant needs and scheduling constraints may require that you select, resequence, or modify the materials in this book. For many groups, verbal presentation of theoretical concepts will be more effective than having the participants read the workbook. After discussing the two pages of questions in Chapter 1 (pp. 4-5) regarding participants' current lifestyle concerns and priorities, the therapist may tailor the agenda and format of subsequent activities accordingly.

A Note for Occupational Therapy Faculty Members and Students

Working with challenging lifestyle issues is an important part of occupational therapy practice. Personal experience with the process of self-assessment and planned change can be a valuable addition to theoretical learning in the classroom.

Assignments that enable students to work in dyads on lifestyle issues of concern to each partner over the course of a semester have been highly productive. Students choose issues that are important to them but are not uncomfortably personal. They gain insight into the complexity of the process of identifying and addressing lifestyle issues and develop sensitive therapeutic skills and an indispensable appreciation for the client experience.

The workbook materials provide a practical structure for collaborative work in dyads. Students identify the element of the Model of Human Occupation most at issue in each situation and use exercises to clarify their concerns. The chapter on change (see p. 71) can be used as a springboard for planning and action.

The instructor should float among dyads during working sessions in order to consult with those encountering difficulties. Brief case presentations at semester's end provide opportunities to solidify learning, celebrate accomplishments, and improve oral reporting skills.

The experiences described above can be comfortably integrated with course material in Psychosocial Dysfunction, Occupational Therapy Theory and Practice, Clinical Reasoning, and Therapeutic Process.

Table of Contents

1.

Introduction

We all have lifestyles—not just those who are rich and famous.

The pattern and performance of one's daily activities weave a fabric of existence that determines the quality of a person's life. *Wellness and Lifestyle Renewal* is a way to gather the cloth of life into one's hands and to rework its design.

Dissatisfaction can be an engine for change. As values and desires are reconsidered, clear goals gradually emerge.

Practical action plans are developed and tried, revised and practiced, until new patterns are established.

Change is a slow and winding path. Life is worth the hike.

Dissatisfaction may have spurred you to begin this *Wellness and Lifestyle Renewal* process. Perhaps long-standing disappointments have bubbled to the surface, or some alteration in circumstances has pressed you to consider a change. It is important to recognize the source and intensity of your dissatisfaction. Pain and trouble can be great motivators. We are most open to new possibilities in times of crisis. On the other hand, stress depletes our energy and resources, sometimes making it difficult to mobilize sustained efforts.

Answer the questions on the next two pages to clarify the purpose of your participation in *Wellness and Lifestyle Renewal*. Reading each section of this book in sequence and completing all of the exercises are recommended. Everyone should begin with Chapter 2, Lifestyles and the Model of Human Occupation. As you identify areas of dissatisfaction in your life, however, you may wish to concentrate your attention on the chapters most relevant for you. The numerals on the second page will guide you to chapters most closely related to questions 1 through 10. When you are satisfied with your exploration of lifestyle components, you may proceed to the chapters (11-13) focused on the change process, self-assessment, and action plans.

Questions

From your perspective, what is a lifestyle?

What is the most important characteristic, issue, or conflict of your current lifestyle?

What do you hope to gain from the *Wellness and Lifestyle Renewal* process?

What question or concern do you have about your participation?

Exercise

Lifestyle Inventory

Relevant Chapters		Strongly Disagree		Neutral		Strongly Agree
3, 4	1. I know clearly what I want to get out of life.	1	2	3	4	5
7, 10	2. I am effective in accomplishing important goals and tasks.	1	2	3	4	5
5, 6	3. I am satisfied with the rhythm and balance of time I spend in work, leisure, chores, and rest.	1	2	3	4	5
4, 5, 10	4. I regularly participate in the activities I enjoy the most.	1	2	3	4	5
4, 7	5. I do a good job of managing my health, home, and finances.	1	2	3	4	5
4, 9	6. I experience a full range of feelings and deal with my emotions well.	1	2	3	4	5
4, 8	7. I have enough intellectual stimulation in my life.	1	2	3	4	5
4, 5, 8	8. I have found meaningful ways to meet my spiritual needs.	1	2	3	4	5
8	9. I am comfortable with the places in which I live, work, recreate, and relax.	1	2	3	4	5
8	10. The relationships and social environments I have chosen are positive and supportive.	1	2	3	4	5

2.

Lifestyles and the Model of Human Occupation

The field of psychology contains competing schools of thought; some emphasize the inner world of thought and feeling, while others stress the importance of behavior alone. But such narrow approaches present only a fragmented view of human psychology unless efforts are made to relate them to functional and experiential dimensions of life.

Wellness and Lifestyle Renewal acknowledges an intimate connection between contemplation and action. Our self-worth depends greatly on the success of our active efforts to influence the world around us. And competent action, in turn, depends upon our inner resources of motivation, planning, and judgment.

The ideas presented in this chapter serve as an orientation to this integrated approach. As an active learner, you will be asked to reflect upon your own life experiences in relation to these concepts.

Reflection

The first and only basis of virtue or a system of right living is the seeking of what is useful to oneself.

Baruch Spinoza (1632-1677)

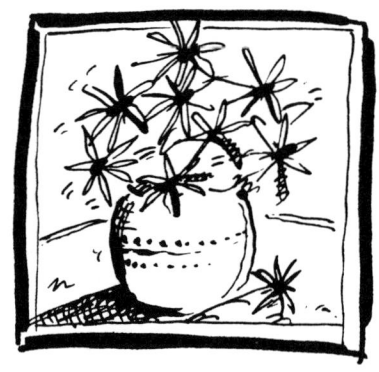

Our lifestyles consist of the things we decide to do each day, the way we do them, and the end results of our efforts in terms of accomplishment and satisfaction. Kielhofner (1985) has developed the Model of Human Occupation, which depicts the human being as an open system that transforms itself and its environment through purposeful action (or occupation)—see Figure 1 on the next page. Each active effort produces feedback for the individual, consisting of both the concrete results of the action and the reactions of other people. This information bolsters or subverts the individual's self-confidence and fosters the refinement of skills and strategies for further action.

In this model, three subsystems—Volition (personal causation, interests, and goals), Habituation (chosen roles and habits), and Performance (skills)— must work together. In other words, our desires must fit with our routines and abilities if we are to succeed, learn, and develop self-confidence. This fit or coordination is called "system organization," and positive results create an upward trajectory of growth and satisfaction for the individual.

For example, a person may have the goal of becoming a biochemist. That desire will be achieved only if the individual possesses both the skills to master scientific material and the study habits necessary to fulfill the role of student. Clearly, problems of "system organization" can take many forms. Another individual may have the ability to study biochemistry but does not believe in his or her effectiveness in this area. This person then sets a career goal to become a baker rather than a biochemist. Of course, neither vocation is intrinsically superior or inferior. But the functional issue involves the congruence or fit between the subsystems in selecting goals, maintaining role-related habit patterns, and producing purposeful actions necessary for success. While work was the focus of the foregoing example, the same dynamics pertain to the performance of chores and leisure occupations as well.

Obviously, the physical and sociocultural environments in which a person functions have an important influence upon his or her opportunities, expectations, and experiences. The role of the environment will be explored in detail later.

The following chapters will describe the elements of the human system. Exercises will help you to reflect upon your own system's characteristics and dynamics.

Figure 1. The Model of Human Occupation

The Model of Human Occupation

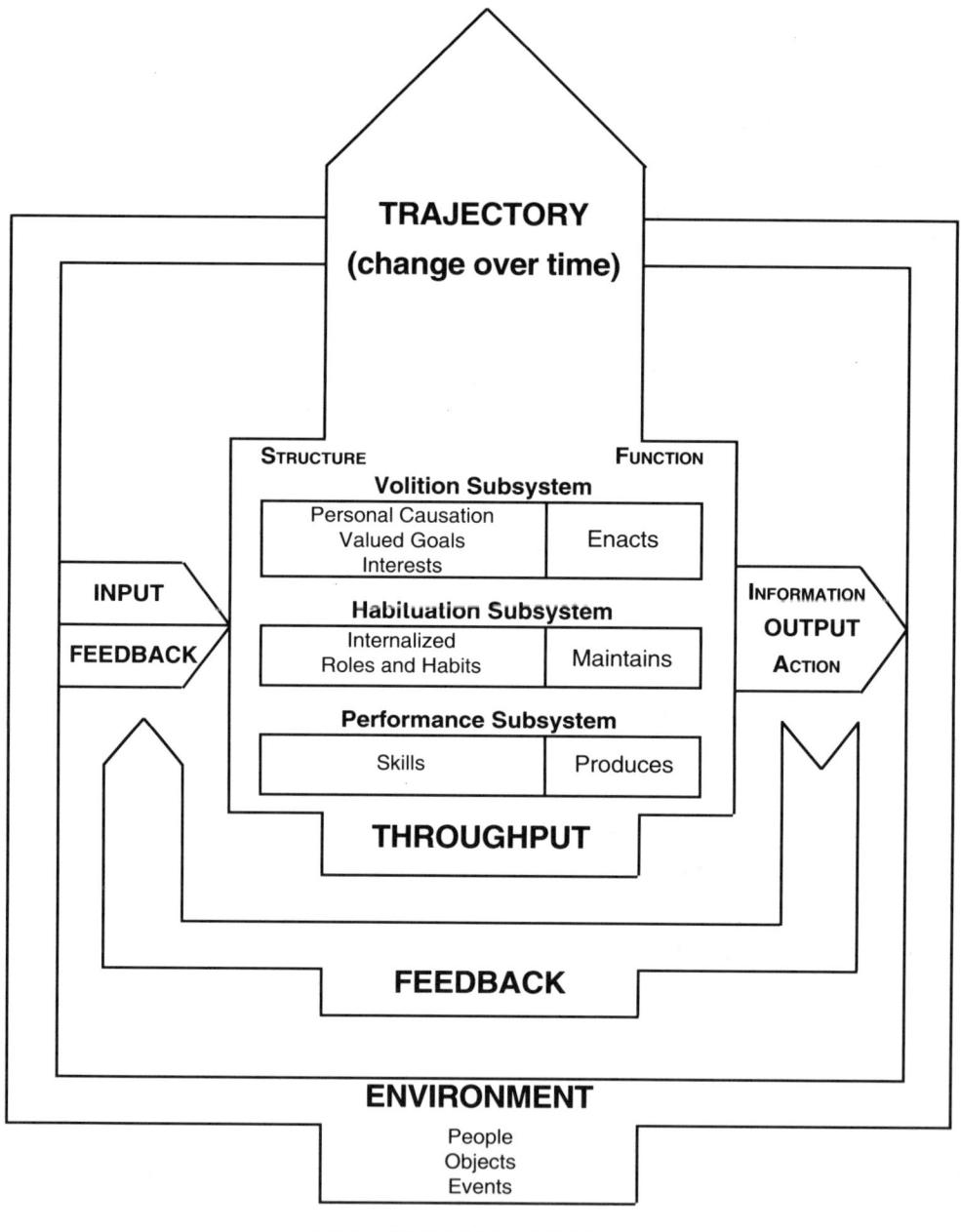

Adapted with permission from Kielhofner, G., & Burke, J. (1980). A model of human occupation, part I: Conceptual framework and content. *American Journal of Occupational Therapy, 34*, 572-581.

3.

Personal Causation

Rejecting Freud's assertion that tension reduction is the overriding goal of human behavior, Robert White, an ego psychologist, developed a "competence model" of human behavior (1971). If our goal is to reduce tension, White asked, why do people go on roller-coaster rides? Why do babies insist upon feeding themselves when more food would find the mouth and less would reach the floor if mom or dad held the spoon? White concluded that we innately strive to explore and master our environments, that we gain a sense of our personal abilities through observing the outcome of our actions. Finally, the quality of our lives is determined by the effectiveness of our actions and by the sense of competence that results.

Personal causation is the belief in one's ability to have a desired impact upon the environment through one's own efforts. Without a realistic and positive sense of personal causation, there is no motivation spurring the human system to act. Some participants enter a *Wellness and Lifestyle Renewal* workshop feeling dissatisfied yet motivated to change in some way. They may also feel frustrated by past failures to address a particular problem. Personal causation in that area, then, is weak. Careful attention should be given to these issues so that internal motivators and obstacles are clearly understood by the participants and the group leader.

Reflections

The world can only be grasped by action, not by contemplation ... The hand is the cutting edge of the mind. Civilization is not a collection of finished artifacts, it is the elaboration of processes. In the end, the march of man is the refinement of the hand in action.

Joseph Bronowski (1980)

The Urge Toward Competence

Human beings possess an innate drive to explore and master the environment. There is joy in being a cause.

Robert White (1971)

Questions

Consider your past efforts to solve problems in your day-to-day life:

As a rule, how thoroughly do you think through and plan for things you wish to do or accomplish? Describe.

Once you know what you want to do, how systematically do you act to accomplish it? Explain.

Does your urge to explore the environment and master new experiences feel strong these days, or has it been weakened by boredom or discouraging experiences? Discuss.

Viktor Frankl was a psychologist imprisoned at Auschwitz during World War II. To cope with this traumatic situation, he studied himself and his fellow inmates. Frankl (1963) discovered that those who could cling to a goal, even the simplest and most mundane, were those who survived psychologically. He concluded that our sense of purpose in life is a most critical resource, since it focuses our efforts and gives meaning to our lives.

Complete the Purpose in Life Test (Crumbaugh, 1968) beginning on page 15 and use the questions on page 19 to reflect upon the sources of meaning in your life.

Exercise

The Purpose in Life Test

For each of the following statements, circle the number that would be most nearly true for you. Note that the numbers always extend from one extreme feeling to its opposite kind of feeling. "Neutral" implies no judgment either way. Try to use this rating as little as possible.

1. I am usually:

1	2	3	4	5	6	7
completely bored			(neutral)		exuberant, enthusiastic	

2. Life to me seems:

7	6	5	4	3	2	1
always exciting			(neutral)		completely routine	

3. In life I have:

1	2	3	4	5	6	7
no goals or aims at all			(neutral)		very clear goals and aims	

4. My personal existence is:

1	2	3	4	5	6	7
utterly meaningless, without purpose			(neutral)		very purposeful and meaningful	

5. Every day is:

7	6	5	4	3	2	1
constantly new and different			(neutral)		exactly the same	

6. If I could choose, I would:

1	2	3	4	5	6	7
prefer never to have been born			(neutral)		like 9 more lives just like this one	

7. After retiring, I would:

7	6	5	4	3	2	1
do some of the exciting things I have always wanted to			(neutral)		loaf completely the rest of my life	

8. In achieving life goals, I have:

1	2	3	4	5	6	7
made no progress whatsoever			(neutral)		progressed to complete fulfillment	

9. My life is:

1	2	3	4	5	6	7
empty, filled only with despair			(neutral)		running over with exciting good things	

10. If I should die today, I would feel that my life has been:

7	6	5	4	3	2	1
very worthwhile			(neutral)		completely worthless	

11. In thinking of my life, I:

1	2	3	4	5	6	7
often wonder why I exist			(neutral)		always see a reason for my being here	

12. As I view the world in relation to my life, the world:

1	2	3	4	5	6	7
completely confuses me			(neutral)		fits meaningfully with my life	

13. I am a:

1	2	3	4	5	6	7
very irresponsible person			(neutral)		very responsible person	

14. Concerning man's freedom to make his own choices, I believe man is:

7	6	5	4	3	2	1
absolutely free to make all life choices			(neutral)		completely bound by limitations of heredity and environment	

15. With regard to death, I am:

7	6	5	4	3	2	1
prepared and unafraid			(neutral)		unprepared and frightened	

16. With regard to suicide, I have

1	2	3	4	5	6	7
thought of it seriously as a way out			(neutral)		never given it a second thought	

17. I regard my ability to find a meaning, purpose, or mission in life as:

7	6	5	4	3	2	1
very great			(neutral)		practically none	

18. My life is:

7	6	5	4	3	2	1
in my hands and I am in control of it			(neutral)		out of my hands and controlled by external factors	

19. Facing my daily tasks is:

7	6	5	4	3	2	1
a source of pleasure and satisfaction			(neutral)		a painful and boring experience	

20. I have discovered:

1	2	3	4	5	6	7
no mission or purpose in life			(neutral)		clear-cut goals and a satisfying life purpose	

To determine your total score, add the numerical value of each of the ratings that you circled.

Your Score: _____

Based upon Viktor Frankl's work, this scale offers feedback about the amount of meaning or existential frustration a person experiences in his or her life. Total scores range from 20 (low purpose) to 140 (high purpose). A score of 108.5 was the norm for a group of college undergraduates; for successful businessmen and professionals, 118.9 (230 subjects).

The Purpose in Life Test is from Crumbaugh, J. (1968). Cross-validation of purpose-in-life test based on Frankl's concepts. *Journal of Individual Psychology, 24*(1), 74-81. Reprinted by permission of the author and the University of Texas Press.

Questions

What observations do you have about your current sense of purpose in life?

What roles and activities provide you with the strongest sense of purpose?

What areas of life leave you feeling most frustrated or empty?

Complete the Internal vs. External Locus of Control exercise (Rotter, 1971), which follows. An explanation of this exercise and a few summary questions appear afterwards.

Exercise

Internal vs. External Control

Please circle 'a' or 'b' for each of the following items, choosing the statement that most closely reflects your attitude or belief.

1. a. Promotions are earned through hard work and persistence.

    <u>b</u>. Making a lot of money is largely a matter of getting the right breaks.

2. a. In my experience I have noticed that there is usually a direct connection between how hard I study and the grades I get.

    <u>b</u>. Many times the reactions of teachers seem haphazard to me.

3. <u>a</u>. Marriage is largely a gamble.

    b. The number of divorces indicates that more and more people are not trying to make their marriages work.

4. <u>a</u>. It is silly to think that one can really change another person's basic attitudes.

    b. When I am right, I can convince others.

5. <u>a</u>. Getting promoted is really a matter of being a little luckier than the next guy.

    b. In our society, a person's future earning power is dependent upon his ability.

6. a. If one knows how to deal with people they are really quite easily led.

    <u>b</u>. I have little influence over the way other people behave.

7. a. In my case, the grades I make are the result of my own efforts; luck has little or nothing to do with it.

    <u>b</u>. Sometimes I feel that I have little to do with the grades I get.

8. a. People like me can change the course of world affairs if we make ourselves heard.

   <u>b.</u> It is only wishful thinking to believe that one can really influence what happens in society at large.

9. <u>a.</u> A great deal that happens to me is probably a matter of chance.

   b. I am the master of my fate.

10. a. Getting along with people is a skill that must be practiced.

    <u>b.</u> It is almost impossible to figure out how to please some people.

This forced choice test indicates whether you tend to believe that rewards in life are the result of your own characteristics or behavior (internal locus of control) or, on the other hand, that these rewards are controlled by luck, fate, or powerful others (external locus of control). One's tendency to believe in internal or external control may affect one's efforts to influence the conditions of one's life, one's way of understanding success and failure, and one's way of viewing personal responsibility.

Compute your score by counting 1 point for each of your answers that was underlined on the test form. A score above 5 indicates that you tend toward an external locus of control while a score below 5 fits with an internal locus of control.

Your Score _____.

The Internal vs. External Control exercise originally appeared in Rotter, J.B. (1971). External control and internal control. *Psychology Today, 5*(1), 42. Reprinted with permission.

Questions

Does your score on the Internal vs. External Control exercise seem to reflect an actual tendency on your part?

How does your internal or external locus of control status affect your way of looking at life?

How does it spur you to or hold you back from making efforts to influence events?

How does it shape the way you deal with issues of responsibility?

4.

Valued Goals and Interests

Our goals and interests develop and change over time. They provide the direction for our actions and the meaning for our efforts. If we lose touch with these beacons of existence, then we may become lost, confused, and even depressed. On the other hand, participating more often in our favorite activities can make us happier human beings.

Each person's goals and interests are shaped in part by social forces and in part by individual preference. As early as 1950, David Riesman described the homogenized conformity that subsumed the behavior of certain social groups. Many suburbanites of the time strove to "keep up with the Joneses" by possessing the same kinds of homes, lawns, cars, and clothing and having the same kinds of careers and leisure interests.

Even without this propensity toward conformity, shared circumstances sometimes shape lifestyles in a similar way. Parents of young children, for example, have many experiences in common: there is never enough time for quiet conversation; an uninterrupted night's sleep is considered a blessing; travel is nearly impossible; and the washing machine seems to run nonstop.

Environments are sometimes created to address the shared lifestyle needs of an entire population—for instance, retirement communities in Florida and Arizona.

However, we may tend to overgeneralize about the lifestyles of certain groups, such as college students, drug addicts, yuppies, gays, single parents, and middle Americans. Although we are strongly influenced by our social groups, life stages, and circumstances, people's lifestyles often express a great deal of individuality. Uniqueness is created by the pursuit of personally determined goals and interests. Like me, you may know a married man who lives in the suburbs and who has recently become a grandfather. The man I know, however, has a pilot's license and an absorbing interest in Kundalini Yoga.

Read the following quotes, which focus on personal goals and interests, and answer the related questions.

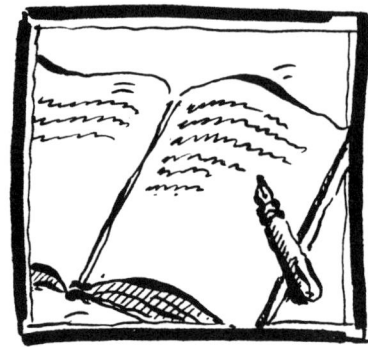

Reflection

Valued goals drive us toward purposeful activity, the use of
our resources of energy, time, interest, and attention to
complete life tasks.

Pat Nuse Clark (1979)

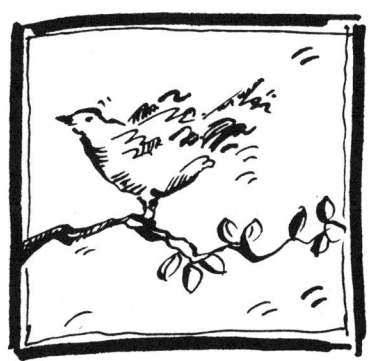

Reflections

Goals create tension systems inside us. These task tensions keep us moving toward our goals until they are achieved (or abandoned) and the tension is released. Uncompleted tasks linger in our minds.

Kurt Lewin (1935)

Short-term goals sustain interest and are guides for action and markers of progress.

Joan Rogers (1982)

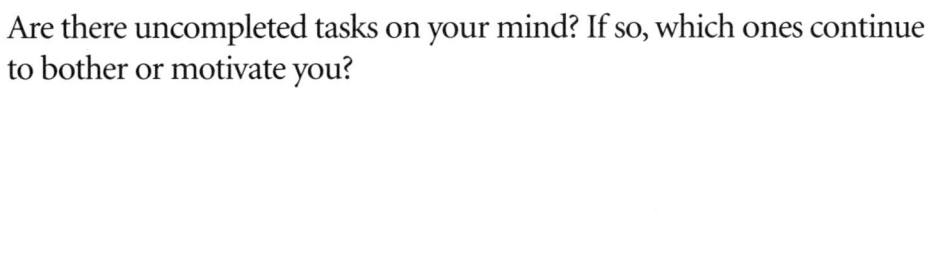

Questions

Are there uncompleted tasks on your mind? If so, which ones continue to bother or motivate you?

Do you tend to notice small achievements toward a long-term goal, or do you simply keep your eyes on the prize? How does this tendency affect you along the way?

Have you abandoned goals prematurely? When have you given up too quickly or easily?

Has it been hard for you to accept defeat and move on? In what instances has this occurred?

Reflection

The mind—all logic—is like the knife—all blade.
It cuts the hand that uses it.

Rabindranath Tagore (1928)

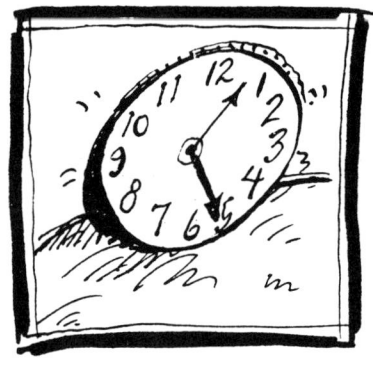

Goals and interests often involve rather concrete and practical matters. Tagore (1928) reminds us, though, that we must look beyond the purely logical and pragmatic to hold life fully in our hands. In the next section, we add spiritual concerns to the physical, emotional, and intellectual elements of life. The spiritual dimension of life has great importance to many Americans. While spirituality is not normally accorded much attention in the Model of Human Occupation, its absence would leave us with an incomplete view of lifestyle issues. These four planes of existence—physical, emotional, intellectual, and spiritual—seem to fit well with a consideration of life goals and interests (Scholem, 1965; Brown, 1971).

Philosophical systems and religious sources as diverse as the Kabalah and Native American religions identify these four planes as central to human existence (Scholem, 1965; Brown, 1971). The planes are commonly conceptualized in a hierarchy of higher to lower concerns—from spiritual to physical.

One may devote great attention to the tasks of a single plane or seek fulfillment in all four equally. No prescription for a satisfying life will be offered here in this regard. One must order the importance of these planes for oneself. Life events may thrust a particular plane to the forefront. Health, emotional stability, learning, and spiritual growth, therefore, are more or less compelling at different times of life. Also, it is clear that items assigned to one plane may impact on another. Finances, for example, involve concrete possessions in the physical plane. Who would deny, though, that money is connected with emotions? If one studies investments and tax laws, then finances enter the intellectual plane as well. The four planes are designed to help us look at important elements of our lifestyle infrastructure. Use these categories flexibly as they best apply to you.

As you read the contents of the four planes on the next page, consider your past and present involvement with each.

The Planes of Existence

Physical Plane

Illness, ailments, and injuries

Nutrition, exercise, and rest

Substance use and abuse

Sexuality

Personal appearance

Finances

Sensory and motor skills

Living environment

Emotional Plane

Range of feelings and moods

Acceptance and expression of feelings
and needs

Giving and receiving love and
emotional support

Control of destructive impulses

Stressful life events

Self-esteem

Intellectual Plane

Work-related study

Leisure reading, interests, projects

Knowledge of current events

Stimulating discussions

Use of community educational
resources

Spiritual Plane

Worship, meditation, and
religious study

Connection with local and
global ecology

Charitable projects,
political/social causes

Relatedness to ancestors, peers,
children, and future generations

Questions

In which planes have you focused most attention?

Which ones have you tended to ignore?

In which planes has growth and satisfaction occurred? Where have you been frustrated?

Think of your time, energy, and attention as quantifiable resources. In what way would you like to shift these resources in order to address physical, emotional, intellectual, or spiritual needs?

Work

Many of our goals and interests involve work, leisure, or chores. All three are important. American culture tends to emphasize work. "Regardless of the form it takes, work represents structure, it provides an outlet for drives, it satisfies both financial needs and familial obligations" (Cori, 1977, p. 283). Mumford (1977) asserts that "in the absence of extended family or caste or clan or religion as a means of social placement, our society relies most heavily on occupation as the means of identifying where people 'belong' in the social structure" (p. 296).

Three major forces are currently impacting on our experience of work and career. First, the economic recession has severely reduced job security and availability for many Americans. Second, many women have joined the work force, offering them new avenues for personal growth and satisfaction, but increasing time and task pressures on mothers, on families, and certainly on single parents who work. Third, Harvey-Krefting (1985) believes that technological change and modern production practices contribute to increasing alienation among workers who do not have opportunities to develop a real sense of craftsmanship or possess a clear connection to the end product of their work.

In assessing your current work satisfaction, reflect upon the following areas. Identify strengths and weaknesses.

Employment and employment potential

Salary and benefits

Responsibility

Advancement

Performance pressure

Work schedule

Work environment (physical and social)

Work content and tasks

Variety and new learning

Consistency and predictability

Supervision and communication

Job security

In thinking about your career, consider whether or not you have:

A clear direction

Appropriate training, credentials, and experiences

Good contacts, supporters, or a mentor

A strategy to move in the direction you have chosen

Leisure

Earning leisure time is one of the great benefits of working. But it can be challenging to create enjoyable leisure. While we have free choice of what to do, we must take all the responsibility for choosing and planning, or we will be twiddling our thumbs in boredom. Some people do not take leisure life seriously since it is "only about having fun."

Reflection

People are often so busy trying to be successful that they forget all about being happy. In a recent study conducted by Reich and Zautra, subjects who followed instructions to increase the frequency of participation in their favorite activities for one month were happier than their counterparts who were instructed not to vary their usual routines.

Diane Swanbrow (1989)

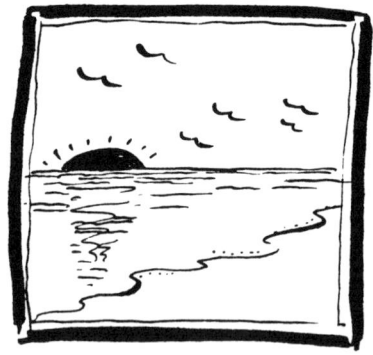

Exercise

Interest Checklist

Complete the Interest Checklist (Matsutsuyu, 1969) below. Notice that spaces separate leisure activities into general categories such as sports, handcrafts, games, intellectual interests, and so on. Use the questions on page 37 to reflect upon your leisure choices.

		CASUAL	STRONG	Pursued in last 3 months			CASUAL	STRONG	Pursued in last 3 months
1.	Golf	❏	❏	❏	25.	Lectures	❏	❏	❏
2.	Football	❏	❏	❏	26.	Reading	❏	❏	❏
3.	Swimming	❏	❏	❏	27.	Computers	❏	❏	❏
4.	Bowling	❏	❏	❏	28.	History	❏	❏	❏
5.	Baseball	❏	❏	❏	29.	Science	❏	❏	❏
6.	Exercise	❏	❏	❏	30.	Politics	❏	❏	❏
7.	Volleyball	❏	❏	❏	31.	Math	❏	❏	❏
8.	Camping	❏	❏	❏	32.	Religion	❏	❏	❏
9.	Tennis	❏	❏	❏					
10.	Scouting	❏	❏	❏	33.	Radio	❏	❏	❏
11.	Basketball	❏	❏	❏	34.	Popular Music	❏	❏	❏
					35.	Classical Music	❏	❏	❏
12.	Sewing	❏	❏	❏	36.	Singing	❏	❏	❏
13.	Needlework	❏	❏	❏	37.	Guitar	❏	❏	❏
14.	Knitting	❏	❏	❏	38.	Concerts	❏	❏	❏
15.	Playing Cards	❏	❏	❏	39.	Piano	❏	❏	❏
16.	Puzzles	❏	❏	❏	40.	Drums	❏	❏	❏
17.	Chess	❏	❏	❏					
18.	Video Games	❏	❏	❏	41.	Gardening	❏	❏	❏
19.	Checkers	❏	❏	❏	42.	Car Repair	❏	❏	❏
20.	Billiards	❏	❏	❏	43.	Manual Arts	❏	❏	❏
21.	Ping Pong	❏	❏	❏	44.	Ironing	❏	❏	❏
22.	Scrabble	❏	❏	❏	45.	Floor Mopping	❏	❏	❏
					46.	Model Building	❏	❏	❏
23.	Languages	❏	❏	❏	47.	Home Repairs	❏	❏	❏
24.	Writing	❏	❏	❏	48.	Woodworking	❏	❏	❏

	CASUAL	STRONG	Pursued in last 3 months			CASUAL	STRONG	Pursued in last 3 months
49. Driving	❑	❑	❑	66. Service Groups		❑	❑	❑
50. Dusting	❑	❑	❑	67. Dancing		❑	❑	❑
51. Jewelry Making	❑	❑	❑					
52. Cooking	❑	❑	❑	68. Movies		❑	❑	❑
53. Leather Work	❑	❑	❑	69. Dramatics		❑	❑	❑
54. Laundry	❑	❑	❑	70. Photography		❑	❑	❑
55. Decorating	❑	❑	❑	71. Painting		❑	❑	❑
56. Shopping	❑	❑	❑	72. Television		❑	❑	❑
57. Hairstyling	❑	❑	❑	73. Ceramics		❑	❑	❑
				74. Mosaics		❑	❑	❑
58. Social Clubs	❑	❑	❑	75. Plays		❑	❑	❑
59. Holidays	❑	❑	❑	76. Clothes		❑	❑	❑
60. Visiting	❑	❑	❑	77. Drawing		❑	❑	❑
61. Barbeques	❑	❑	❑	78. Collecting		❑	❑	❑
62. Traveling	❑	❑	❑	79. Pets		❑	❑	❑
63. Parties	❑	❑	❑					
64. Conversation	❑	❑	❑	80. Other _____		❑	❑	❑
65. Dating	❑	❑	❑	81. Other _____		❑	❑	❑

Adapted with permission from Matsutsuyu, J. (1969). The interest checklist. *American Journal of Occupational Therapy, 23,* 323-328.

Questions

Does your current range of interests seem broad or narrow?

Are you comfortable with this range of interests?

What activity and which category are your favorites?

How often do you engage in your preferred occupations?

What obstacles limit your pursuit of leisure enjoyment?

What is most important to you about the way you spend free time?

Chores

Chores can be defined as "physical or mental activity directed toward the maintenance of an individual's personal self and living space. It includes activities such as shopping, meal preparation, laundry, personal hygiene, housecleaning, driving a car or using public transportation, using the telephone and paying bills" (Schwartzberg, 1982, p. 2). People vary greatly in the time and effort they devote to these tasks and in the value they place upon them. Individuals, roommates, families, organizations, and even whole communities and countries make decisions about the standards with which such tasks will be completed and about the assignment of these responsibilities. In thinking about your own chores, consider the following:

Did you participate in family chores as a child? How did this experience shape your current attitude and approach?

How comfortable are you with the way chores are distributed among those with whom you live and with whom you work?

Questions
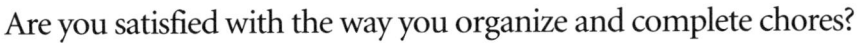

Are you satisfied with the way you organize and complete chores?

Are you comfortable with the standards you and significant others set for completion of chores?

5.

Internalized Roles

The study of human development was considered a pediatric science until about 1970. Physical and psychological development were thought to progress intensively in a stage-ordered fashion through adolescence and to tail off in the settled sameness of adulthood.

Current theories of development dispute this view. Theorists such as Lidz (1968), Sheehey (1974), and Kohlberg (1968) have launched investigations into the developmental challenges of adult life. Men and women of our era have experimented widely with career changes, family configurations, retirement options, health habits, and spiritual quests. In sum, for many people, adulthood today possesses a great richness of self-determined possibilities.

So many possibilities and such high expectations, however, contain advantages and disadvantages. As human beings, we are limited in the options we can exercise. We have only so much energy and time at our disposal. We have responsibilities to others that may not be cast aside without consequence.

In this chapter, we will look at the map of internalized expectations for life that we each possess and at the roles that we occupy. And in the following chapter, we will examine the way we spend time in an effort to fulfill our chosen roles.

A map is drawn by a map maker. We, too, may see our inner maps illuminated by self-awareness and take up eraser and pen on our own behalf.

Reflection

In our minds we each have a cognitive map, a complex set of
expectations for how life will be as we progress through it.
Great deviations from the pattern of this map can cause
confusion and disappointment.

J. R. Taplin (1971)

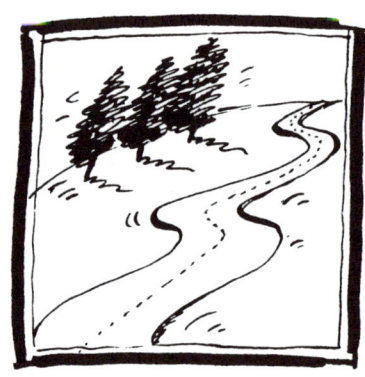

The roles that we assume create a framework that structures our lives. In developing a lifestyle, it is critical to direct our efforts toward fulfilling life roles with which we strongly identify. Some people try to cover all the bases, to enjoy the rewards of all the possible roles (see the list below). They cannot succeed. Our current American culture, it seems, may foster this unrealistic expectation, and thereby program us for disappointment. For example, a woman in a recent *Wellness and Lifestyle Renewal* workshop complained that she felt compelled to stop reading women's magazines. "They suggest," she said, "that I should have a fast-track career; be a super-mom, an exciting lover, a supportive spouse, a gourmet cook, and an intimate friend; and pursue stimulating hobbies in order to feel satisfied with my life." The woman felt frazzled and incomplete.

In general, we experience role dysfunction when we are seriously over- or undercommitted to roles. While some roles are prescribed for us by society, we still have a wide range of choices. Read about role dysfunctions on the next page with an eye toward your own role selection patterns, and then complete the Role Checklist (Oakley, 1984) to identify past satisfactions and disappointments as well as desires for the future.

Great Expectations: A Pantheon of Roles

To be, to have, to give, to experience, to accomplish:

- Exciting, meaningful, successful career(s)
- Terrific love life
- Committed long-term relationship
- Involved, responsible parent and/or child
- Rich friendships
- Interesting, varied leisure life
- Well-decorated and maintained home
- Service to community
- Spiritual growth
- Travel

Role Dysfunction

Overcommitted	Undercommitted
• Too many roles	• Too few roles
• Role performance expectations too high	• Role performance expectations too low
• Static, inflexible roles	• Role hopping and role dabbling due to weakly chosen and established roles or too many roles
• Single role takeover	

Exercise

Role Checklist

Name: _____ Age: _____ Date: _____

Sex: ❑ Male ❑ Female   Are you retired? ❑ Yes ❑ No

Marital Status: ❑ Single ❑ Married ❑ Separated ❑ Divorced ❑ Widowed

The purpose of this checklist is to identify the major roles in your life. The checklist, which is divided into two parts, presents 10 roles and defines each one.

Part One

Beside each role indicate by checking the appropriate column if you performed the role in the past, if you presently perform the role, and if you plan to perform the role in the future. You may check more than one column for each role. For example, if you volunteered in the past, do not volunteer at the present, but plan to in the future, you would check the past and future columns.

Role	Past	Present	Future
STUDENT: Attending school on a part-time or full-time basis.			
WORKER: Part-time or full-time paid employment.			
VOLUNTEER: Donating services, at least once a week, to a hospital, school, community, political campaign, and so forth.			
CARE GIVER: Responsibility, at least once a week, for the care of someone, such as a child, spouse, relative, or friend.			
HOME MAINTAINER: Responsibility, at least once a week, for the upkeep of the home, such as housecleaning or yardwork.			
FRIEND: Spending time or doing something, at least once a week, with a friend.			
FAMILY MEMBER: Spending time or doing something, at least once a week, with a family member, such as a child, spouse, parent, or other relative.			
RELIGIOUS PARTICIPANT: Involvement, at least once a week, in groups or activities affiliated with one's religion (excluding worship).			
HOBBYIST/AMATEUR: Involvement, at least once a week, in a hobby or amateur activity, such as sewing, playing a musical instrument, woodworking, sports, the theater, or participation in a club or team.			
PARTICIPANT IN ORGANIZATIONS: Involvement, at least once a week, in organizations, such as the American Legion, National Organization for Women, Parents Without Partners, Weight Watchers, and so forth.			
OTHER: A role not listed that you have performed, are presently performing, and/or plan to perform. Write the role on the line below and check the appropriate column(s). _____			

Part Two

The same roles are listed below. Next to each role, check the column that best indicates how valuable or important the role is to you. Answer for each role, even if you have never performed or do not plan to perform the role.

Role	Not At All Valuable	Somewhat Valuable	Very Valuable
STUDENT: Attending school on a part-time or full-time basis.			
WORKER: Part-time or full-time paid employment.			
VOLUNTEER: Donating services, at least once a week, to a hospital, school, community, political campaign, and so forth.			
CARE GIVER: Responsibility, at least once a week, for the care of someone, such as a child, spouse, relative, or friend.			
HOME MAINTAINER: Responsibility, at least once a week, for the upkeep of the home, such as housecleaning or yardwork.			
FRIEND: Spending time or doing something, at least once a week, with a friend.			
FAMILY MEMBER: Spending time or doing something, at least once a week, with a family member, such as a child, spouse, parent, or other relative.			
RELIGIOUS PARTICIPANT: Involvement, at least once a week, in groups or activities affiliated with one's religion (excluding worship).			
HOBBYIST/AMATEUR: Involvement, at least once a week, in a hobby or amateur activity, such as sewing, playing a musical instrument, woodworking, sports, the theater, or participation in a club or team.			
PARTICIPANT IN ORGANIZATIONS: Involvement, at least once a week, in organizations, such as the American Legion, National Organization for Women, Parents Without Partners, Weight Watchers, and so forth.			
OTHER: A role not listed that you have performed, are presently performing, and/or plan to perform. Write the role on the line below and check the appropriate column(s). _____			

Adapted from Oakley, F. (1984). *The role checklist*. National Institutes of Health, Department of Rehabilitation Medicine, Occupational Therapy Service. Reprinted with permission of the author.

6.

Habit Patterns

Some things in life are best done on automatic pilot. Washing, dressing, grooming, and getting breakfast are accomplished by many of us while our minds are in an early morning fog. A robot-like routine carries us through our morning regimen at a good clip despite the fog, without the necessity of careful attention.

Habits are formed by repetition; we practice the same set of tasks over and over again until they no longer require a great deal of conscious control. A great pianist, for instance, technically masters a piece long before the night of the concert. And he or she does so by bringing to bear the work habits of a professional musician—namely, 6 to 8 hours of practice per day. In effect, habits maintain occupational performance.

Occupational habit patterns can have a positive or negative effect on one's lifestyle. A teenager, for instance, may develop the habit of talking on the phone with friends for long hours every evening. Her social life progresses well, but her grades in high school may plunge as a result.

By nature, habits can be difficult to change. Yet we must be flexible enough to change our habits as circumstances require. For example, a man who always described himself as a night person found that two weeks into a new job that began at 7 am he had to change his motto to "early to bed and early to rise" in order to survive.

The way we organize time on a daily and weekly basis is at the core of the habits and routines we follow. We have only 24 hours to use each day. We must keep appointments, provide a pace to our day, and hold in perspective our past, present, and future. While many people feel that they have time on their hands, others are always trying to catch up. I met a friend in his 40s for lunch during a recent weekend. While he was on time, he complained that he had had to drive 75 mph to make the appointment. He then admitted that he lives his entire life at that same speed, rushing and out of breath, unable to stop and smell the roses. In contrast, when asked why she had never learned to use the microwave oven that came with her condominium, a retired woman replied that she is in no hurry. Defrosting and cooking food "the old way," she stated, are activities that fit well with the gentle rhythms of her day.

In his book, *Time Wars* (1987), Jeremy Rifkin takes a historical view of our use and understanding of time, a precious commodity of human life. He sees a trend away from biologically and ecologically based rhythms of life. Before the Industrial Revolution's maxim, "time is money," agrarian societies lived by the seasons. People tilled, harvested, and rested as nature's rhythms suggested, waking with the sun and sleeping with the darkness. Historically, many societies have balanced time use more heavily toward leisure than we do today. The Romans reportedly celebrated about 200 feast days a year (although their slaves probably did not get these days off). The Benedictine monks invented the idea of a routine daily schedule in the 6th century in response to their fear that idle hands would do the Devil's work. They programmed themselves to be busy all through the day and invented a clock in the 13th century to better organize their efforts. In the 1990s, according to Rifkin, we are developing a computer culture of nano-second time in which efficiency and speed in transactions are the ascendant values. Mastery, Rifkin believes, dominates empathy in our view of ourselves, our interactions with others, our work, and our use of time—much to our detriment as human beings.

Read the following quotes, and complete the exercises to enrich your perspective about the way you are handling time, your greatest resource.

Reflections

The secret of life is enjoying the passing of time.

James Taylor (1978)

Temporal Balance

Activities provide an organizing structure for the use of one's time and create a rhythm to life.

Each person creates a unique pattern of work, leisure, chores, and rest on a day-to-day basis. The balance and interplay of these elements profoundly affect the health of the individual.

Effective planning and performance of prescribed and chosen activities determines the quality of one's life as well as one's identity in society.

Adolph Meyer (1922)

Reflection

In Support of Idle Leisure and Play

Have we become enslaved by the weekend? . . . The lack of carelessness in our recreation, the sense of obligation to get things right, and the emphasis on protocol and decorum do represent an enslavement of a kind. People used to 'play' tennis; now they 'work' on their backhand.

Witold Rybczynski (1991)

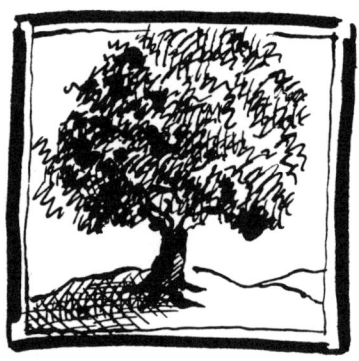

Exercise

Activities Wheel

Complete two Activities Wheel exercises, one for a typical weekday and another for a typical weekend day. Analyze your work/play balance at the bottom of each form.

Each segment of the wheel below stands for one hour of your day. For each hour, write the name of the activity you are doing during that time on a typical day. Use one pie for a typical weekday and another for a typical weekend day.

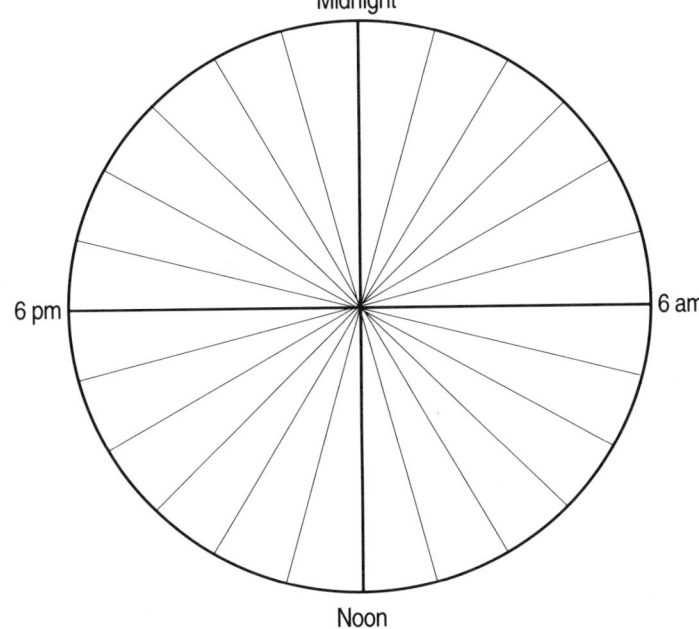

Typical Weekday

Midnight

6 pm

6 am

Noon

ANALYSIS

Rest and Relaxation

How many hours do you spend sleeping? _____

How many hours do you spend resting? _____

How many hours do you spend relaxing, doing something just because you enjoy it? _____

Total: _____

Responsibilities

How many hours do you spend fulfilling responsibilities to others (job, childcare, homemaking, meetings, etc.)? _____

How many hours do you spend on self-maintenance tasks (dressing, grooming, meals, chores, medical appointments, etc.)? _____

Total: _____

Compare the two totals to consider your current work/play balance.

Each segment of the wheel below stands for one hour of your day. For each hour, write the name of the activity you are doing during that time on a typical weekend day.

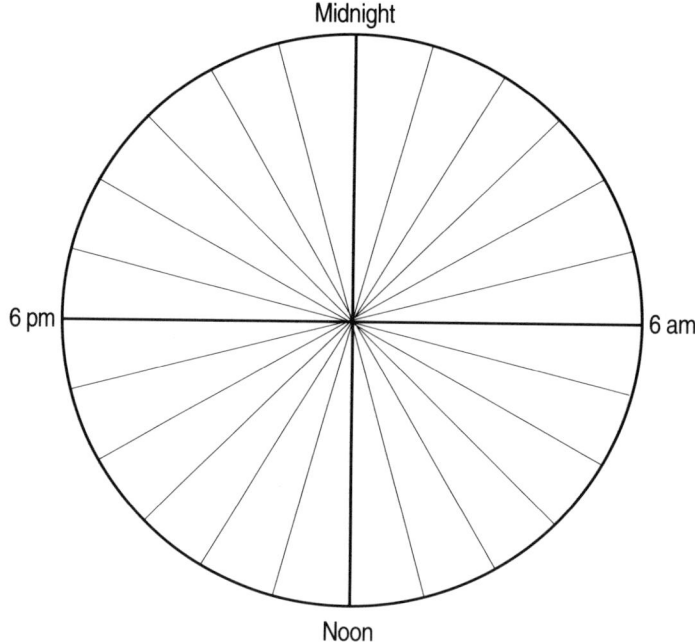

Typical Weekend Day

Midnight

6 pm

6 am

Noon

ANALYSIS

Rest and Relaxation

How many hours do you spend sleeping? _____

How many hours do you spend resting? _____

How many hours do you spend relaxing, doing something just because you enjoy it? _____

Total: _____

Responsibilities

How many hours do you spend fulfilling responsibilities to others (job, childcare, homemaking, meetings, etc.)? _____

How many hours do you spend on self-maintenance tasks (dressing, grooming, meals, chores, medical appointments, etc.)? _____

Total: _____

Compare the two totals to consider your current work/play balance.

Exercise

Activities Configuration

On this form, write the name of the activity you perform at each hour of a typical weekday. Then, rate your performance, enjoyment, and benefit gained in each activity by writing a "+" (positive) or a "–" (negative) in the spaces provided.

Time	Activity	Performance	Enjoyment	Benefit	Comments
6 am					
7					
8					
9					
10					
11					
noon					
1 pm					
2					
3					
4					
5					
6					
7					
8					
9					
10					
11					
midnite					
1 am					
2					
3					
4					
5					
6					

Questions

Having completed the Activities Wheel and Activities Configuration exercises, consider the following questions:

Are you comfortable with your current balance of responsibilities and relaxation—the interplay of work, leisure, chores, and rest?

Does your day proceed at a reasonable pace? Describe.

Which activities generate positive and negative experiences for you? To what extent does your day include positive events?

Do you spend enough time with others and enough time alone?

Do your habit patterns and use of time enable you to fulfill the life roles that are important to you? Explain.

Would you like your typical day to be spent differently in some way? If so, what would you change?

7.

Skills

While personal causation and goals motivate us to action, and role-related habit patterns organize our efforts, *skills* produce occupational behavior. Our ability to carry out our wishes in life is ultimately controlled by the skills that we possess. Human beings develop an incredible range of skills through a life-long process of exploration, imitation, and repetition (Kielhofner, 1985). Even the simplest of skills, such as throwing a ball, requires the coordination of sensory, motor, and cognitive capacities.

We have all heard the adage, "You can't teach an old dog new tricks." Your own lifestyle renewal, however, may require that you learn new skills, enact new roles, accomplish new goals, and pursue new interests. In her exploration of human development, Llorens (1974) insists that we are able to learn and grow throughout the life span by purposeful application of activities with the support and stimulation of relationships. Today's vital senior citizens and the wealth of their accomplishments provide ample evidence that Llorens' assertion is correct.

Mastering new skills, though, means that you must be prepared to tolerate some uncomfortable feelings, including helplessness, dependency, fear of failure, and frustration. While learning can be exciting as well, the above discomforts are a familiar part of the process. You will need patience, playfulness, determination, time, tools, and support in order to succeed. Finally, you must know yourself well enough to measure your desires against a realistic appraisal of your abilities and opportunities.

Questions

Are your skills generally sufficient to accomplish the goals you set for yourself? Describe.

How well do you tolerate the discomforts involved in learning a challenging new skill?

Is there a skill you have mastered as an adult that required real perseverance on your part? What helped you through?

8.
Physical and Social Environments

Human beings develop by a process of mutual accommodation between themselves and their surroundings (Bronfenbrenner, 1979). Each person exists in many environments consisting of people, objects, and events. According to Bandura (1977), "individuals who regard their behavior so highly that the reactions of their associates have no effect on their self-evaluation are rare indeed" (p. 149).

In her functional assessment of children, Lyons (1984) noticed discrepancies between what kids could do independently and what they could do with minor assistance or instruction at critical points. Likewise, our friends, relatives, and co-workers may support and assist us to draw upon tenuous, new abilities emerging within us. But they may also ignore or oppose our efforts to grow.

The life-spaces we choose for work, home, and leisure also influence our performance within them. For example, a large, pleasantly decorated, and well-stocked kitchen with good counter space and appropriate appliances may encourage us to cook, while a less comfortable kitchen may discourage us. In great measure (and according to our means), we are able to select and design our social and physical environments. Although people respond to social, political, economic, and cultural pressure, they are also able to make many of their own decisions regarding their surroundings and lifestyles. Aaron Beck (1976), a pioneer of cognitive methods, said that "the wise person is able to extract the sound principles from the thick brew of his cultural heritage and to ignore the residue of fallacious notions, myths, and superstitions" (p. 13). It is essential that we clearly understand the ways in which we and our environments fit and conflict; if choices and compromises must be made between our lifestyle goals and our surroundings, we will approach these with our eyes wide open.

Read the quotes on page 58 and answer the questions that follow. Consider the impact of the environmental choices that you have made.

Reflections

The Environment

The environments in which we live, work, and play have profound effects upon us. The people, objects, and events in these environments must *arouse* us enough to avoid boredom, but not so much as to cause extreme anxiety. The *performance demands* made upon us by our environments must fit with our skills and competencies if we are to do well. They must match our *values* and *interests* as well, if we are to feel satisfied.

Roann Barris (1982)

Emergent skills are awakened and accessed by cuing, support, and collaboration.

Barbara Lyons (1984)

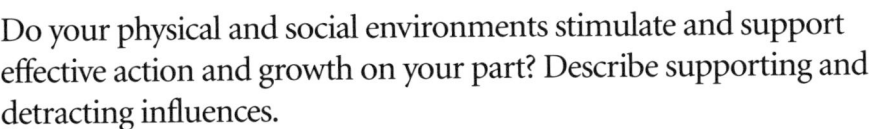 Questions

Do your physical and social environments stimulate and support effective action and growth on your part? Describe supporting and detracting influences.

What individuals are likely to be your strongest supporters in your efforts to change? Who is likely to interfere?

9.

Feedback and Throughput

Gail and Jay Fidler (1978) have stated that human beings formulate objectives, strive toward them, and then evaluate the outcome of their efforts. Each person performs these steps in an individualized way, with positive, negative, or mixed results. It is essential to be realistic in our self-appraisals. But we must avoid being too quick to blame ourselves when things go wrong. Fayans and Maehr (1980) have identified the effect of certain kinds of thinking upon perfomance. From their research, they concluded that the tendency to attribute success to one's ability, while blaming one's failure on inadequate effort, poor instruction, or other external factors, helps people to persevere in the face of frustrating setbacks.

In the Model of Human Occupation, the way one understands or processes feedback from the environment is called "throughput." If one is overly critical or self-congratulatory in response to feedback, system dysfunction may develop. A young artist, for example, may see only the flaws in her work and disregard the praise of others as not genuine. She may become discouraged and turn away from artistic pursuits. On the other hand, a man in his twenties wanted to quit his job as a legal assistant and "go out on his own" after his boss expressed mild enthusiasm for a practical idea he had for improving office efficiency.

Feedback and throughput clearly influence subsequent occupational goals and efforts. All of us have personalities and personal histories that skew our perception in particular areas.

Answer the questions about your learning and self-evaluation process. They will draw your attention to the filter through which you perceive your own performance and the feedback of others.

Reflection

Action is both the product of a mental image that sets the objective and the creator of a mental image . . . including the refinement of strategies and evaluation of the achievement.

Gail and Jay Fidler (1978)

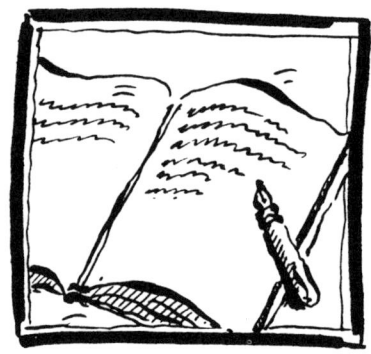

In evaluating your performance, do you tend to be accurate, overly critical, or unrealistically positive?

How well do you learn from mistakes in refining your strategies?

Identify and discuss some specific examples from your past experiences.

Self-Evaluation:

Learning from Experience:

10.

Output and System Trajectory

Nothing Succeeds Like Success

One's occupational efforts (output) profoundly affect the overall direction of change (trajectory) of one's human system. Brewster Smith (1974) used the images of upward and downward spirals of activity to describe this trajectory. In an upward spiral, the person is launched with a sense of self-confidence and is quite willing to take risks. Trials produce errors, but they produce successes as well. And with experience, a person learns and develops skills, and the frequency of his or her success increases. The upward spiral leads to a generalized sense of hopefulness about the future. Smith saw this process as a spiral because of its tendency to build upon itself in an ongoing, positive way. As Joan Rogers (1982, p. 709), an occupational therapy theorist, summarized, "Repeated application of this sequence—of thinking, doing, and evaluating—leads to mastery. By mastering some things, we develop a sense of competence as well as technical skill. Perceived competence leads to an image of the self as a doer. It allows us to say with confidence, 'I can do it. I can achieve.'"

The downward spiral is just the opposite. Launched with a sense of doubt and an expectation of failure, one makes few efforts, learns little, and is unable to build a base of successful experiences. Failures seem devastating, causing the person to feel pessimistic about his or her ability to shape the future.

"Learned helplessness" is an extreme example of the downward spiral. Martin Seligman, a psychologist, studied rats on an electrified grid. When he turned on the current, the rats jumped off to avoid the shock. When Seligman put up a barrier that prevented them from escaping, the rats quickly just laid down on the grid, making no further efforts to escape. They had learned a helpless pattern of behavior. Seligman believed that people can become depressed and helpless like the rats when their efforts have been repeatedly thwarted.

Luckily, a downward spiral can often be turned around by a series of small successes. As Loeb, Beck, and Diggory (1971) have demonstrated, concrete accomplishments can improve a discouraged person's self-esteem, elevate hopes and expectations, and energize further task performances.

There are times in life when one's feelings or values have not yet shifted enough to permit a new action or pattern of behavior to succeed. Efforts to act may only generate conflict or create feelings of failure. Anyone who has attempted to quit smoking before he or she was emotionally prepared to do so has experienced this phenomenon.

On the other hand, we must sometimes act or we will be waiting forever to feel ready. Trying my first front flip from a diving board was just such a situation for me. I concentrated and envisioned the form of the dive; I loosened up my body by bouncing on the board. But eventually, and despite my fears, I had to take the leap. After the first attempt, even though the dive was a mess, my fears diminished. On subsequent tries, my performance improved. Sometimes we can take action, and our feelings will follow! It is important when facing a new challenge to decide whether it is a time to work with feelings and values or a time for action.

Read the following quotes to review the ideas that have been presented. Then answer the questions about your upward and downward spirals that follow.

Reflection

The Upward Spiral

- Believes in own effectiveness

- Seeks opportunities and makes efforts

- Becomes more confident in response to successes

- Gains knowledge and skill through active effort
(making further successes more likely)

- Develops respect for self and hopeful attitude toward future

Brewster Smith (1974)

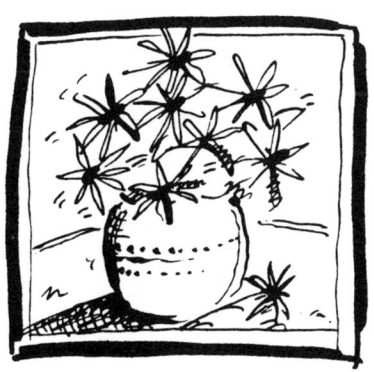

Reflections

Learned Helplessness

Continual thwarting of efforts can lead to a state of depression and learned helplessness, in which the individual no longer tries.

Martin Seligman (1975)

If one's degree of mastery is insufficient, he or she will not be able to handle the stresses of daily living. The individual then becomes more vulnerable to intrapsychic and interpersonal disorganization.

Margot Howe and Anne Briggs (1982)

Reflection

Following successful performance on a task, the *mood, self-esteem, expectation of further success,* and *subsequent task performance*—all improved among members of a depressed group.

A. Loeb, A. Beck, and J. Diggory (1971)

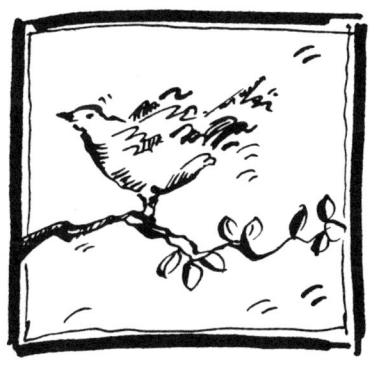

Questions

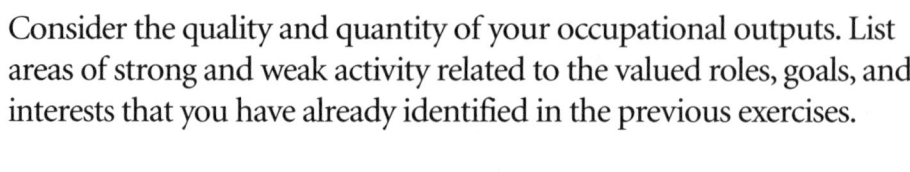

Consider the quality and quantity of your occupational outputs. List areas of strong and weak activity related to the valued roles, goals, and interests that you have already identified in the previous exercises.

Are you currently involved in an upward or downward spiral? What started you moving in your current direction?

Is there an important issue about which you have become too discouraged to continue trying? Explain.

11.

The Change Process and Occupational Adaptation

Finally, we approach the gates of change. It is neither quick nor simple to pass through them because there are obstacles to overcome and dangers to avoid. This chapter offers conceptual and practical tools for change that will help you progress through doubt and fantasy to realistic desire, orderly plans, and systematic actions.

While you may accomplish only a single change in this context, you will have established a method for change. Unlike other animals, human beings have the capacity to remember past experience, to imagine the future, and to create tools with which to meet the challenges of life. By completing this introduction to *Wellness and Lifestyle Renewal*, you will imagine new futures and bear the tools to create them.

Reflection

The most significant distinction between adequate functioning and dysfunction is the degree to which a system (individual, family, society, etc.) is either able to generate change by itself or else is caught in a Game Without End.

Paul Watzlawick, John Weakland, and Richard Fisch (1974)

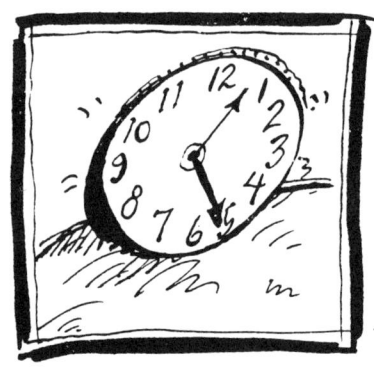

Exercise

What positive changes have you already caused to occur in your way of living? How did you bring each of these changes about?

Changes	Methods

The following quotes emphasize the difficulties of the change process. While we may feel motivated to change, the devil that we know is often more comfortable than the devil that we don't. Fear and conflict can accompany even the most positive changes. And the process is slow. The "quick fix," so highly valued in American culture, is elusive when it comes to personal change and growth. Diligence and patience are both required. Being dissatisfied with the way things are does not mean one possesses a clear vision of a better way, however. Uncertainty must be tolerated and fantasy encouraged in order to discover a proper direction. Once the path of change has been established, one must have clear, short-term goals to provide stepping stones toward the desired end result. In their book on security and change, Nena and George O'Neill (1974, p. 238) state, "While most of the conditions for creativity require a suspension of control, an openness to the inner areas of the self, the last and most important [condition] is using our will to put what we have discovered into action."

While you are reviewing the challenges of the change process and the tools for change listed at the end of this section, consider the following questions:

Which aspects of the change process will be most difficult for you?

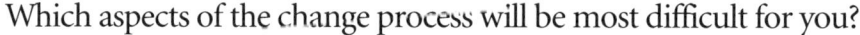

What kind of support and encouragement will help you to overcome the difficulties you anticipate?

Which parts of the change process will come easily for you?

Reflection

Five Realities of the Change Process

1) Change is generally resisted by persons and groups.

2) Change is generally feared by persons and groups.

3) Lasting change only occurs within a context of change.

4) Real change occurs from within outward.

5) Change, to be real and lasting, must be slow and gradual.

George Eastman (c. 1987)

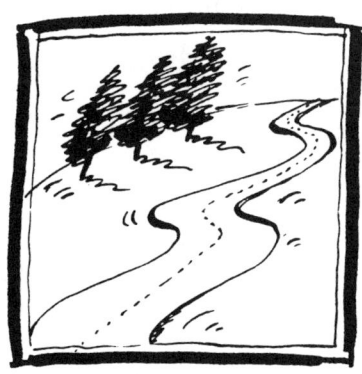

Reflections

The faith waiting in the heart of a seed promises a miracle of life which it cannot prove at once.

Rabindranath Tagore (1928)

Whoever too hastily catches at certainties shall end in doubts, as he who seasonably withholds his judgment shall arrive at certainties.

Francis Bacon (1605)

Reflections

Human freedom involves our capacity to pause between stimulus and response and, in that pause, to choose the one response toward which we wish to throw our weight.

R. May (1978)

Spinoza says that you must fix your attention on a desired virtue, and you will thus tend to acquire it.

H. Wolfson (1950)

Reflections

Worrying is a form of coping behavior when it helps us to prepare and rehearse for difficult situations.

David Hamburg and John Adams (1967)

Fantasy (withdrawal from reality) is necessary for creative problem-solving in preparing for new adaptive efforts.

Heinz Hartmann (1958)

Change involves a challenging interplay between the person and his or her surroundings. Freud (1930) labelled efforts to change oneself as "autoplastic" and efforts to change the environment as "alloplastic." Hartmann (1958) saw both as necessary for adaptation to succeed.

Watzlawick, Weakland, and Fisch (1974) observed that people often fail to change despite energetic efforts. In fact, a person's efforts to solve a problem often create new problems or make the original problem worse. At worst, increasing effort to solve a problem only succeeds in digging a deeper hole for the parties involved, creating "A Game Without End." These authors determined that some changes require only more of something—more effort, more speed, more repetition. One could become more physically fit, for example, by performing aerobic exercises more often, for longer lengths of time, and at an increased level of exertion. This is First Order Change. The process can be likened to stepping harder on the accelerator of an automobile.

In contrast, other changes can only be accomplished by transforming the situation or participants in some way. One must shift gears rather than merely press down on the accelerator. This is Second Order Change. For example, a person having a nightmare may run, hide, fight, or jump off a cliff to escape, but none of these actions ends the nightmare. The only way out of the dream is to make a change from sleeping to waking, an altogether different state of being. Second Order Change requires novel solutions that step outside the usual rules and parameters governing the situation at hand. My wife and I, for example, struggled for months to get our son, then six years old, to eat his dinner. We nagged, cajoled, offered desserts as incentives, all in vain. He insisted that he didn't like the food. Finally, we shifted gears and asked him to list his favorite foods. We agreed to make him dinners selected from the list. Thankfully, his choices were all easy to prepare. Sure enough, our son regained his appetite and dinnertime became a more pleasant family occasion. Second Order Change!

As you begin to formulate a change you wish to make, consider whether First or Second Order Change is required. Review the Tools of Change on the next page to identify the resources at your disposal.

Reflection

Lifestyle Renewal Tools of Change

Disruption and Dissatisfaction

Belief in Own Efficacy

Creative Vision

Risk

Manageable Goals

Concrete Tasks

Realistic Performance Appraisal

Environmental Support

Energy and Endurance

Kielhofner, Barris, and Watts (1982) have described a series of four steps through which one must pass in order to change long-standing habits. The existing habit pattern must be recognized and its inadequacy accepted (Invalidation). Challenging the status quo requires that risks be taken to generate new ways of acting (Exploration). Through trial and error, a new pattern of behavior is chosen (Innovation). Finally, the new pattern becomes routine through practice over time (Habituation).

With respect to a change you are considering or making, at what stage of the habit change process are you currently working?

Reflection

Habit Change Process

Invalidation
(challenge)

Exploration
(risk)

Innovation
(choice)

Habituation
(practice)

Gary Kielhofner, Roann Barris, and Janet Watts (1982)

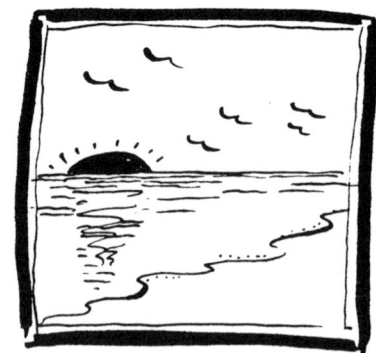

As previously defined, a person's occupational status is his or her degree of life satisfaction derived from the performance of work, leisure, chores, and rest in a temporal pattern that fits the values, needs, and future goals of the individual, while at the same time meeting societal expectations.

According to Rosenfeld (1989), occupational adaptation (change) is stimulated by internal dissatisfaction or by external events, as shown below in Figure 2. These disruptions create strong feelings and mobilize the person to action. They may also crystalize important personal, familial, and developmental issues and conflicts that have been lurking beneath the surface. Disruption leads to a novel and clear recognition of intricate occupational patterns and ecological configurations that are woven into the fabric of life. With options open before him or her,

Figure 2. Occupational Adaptation

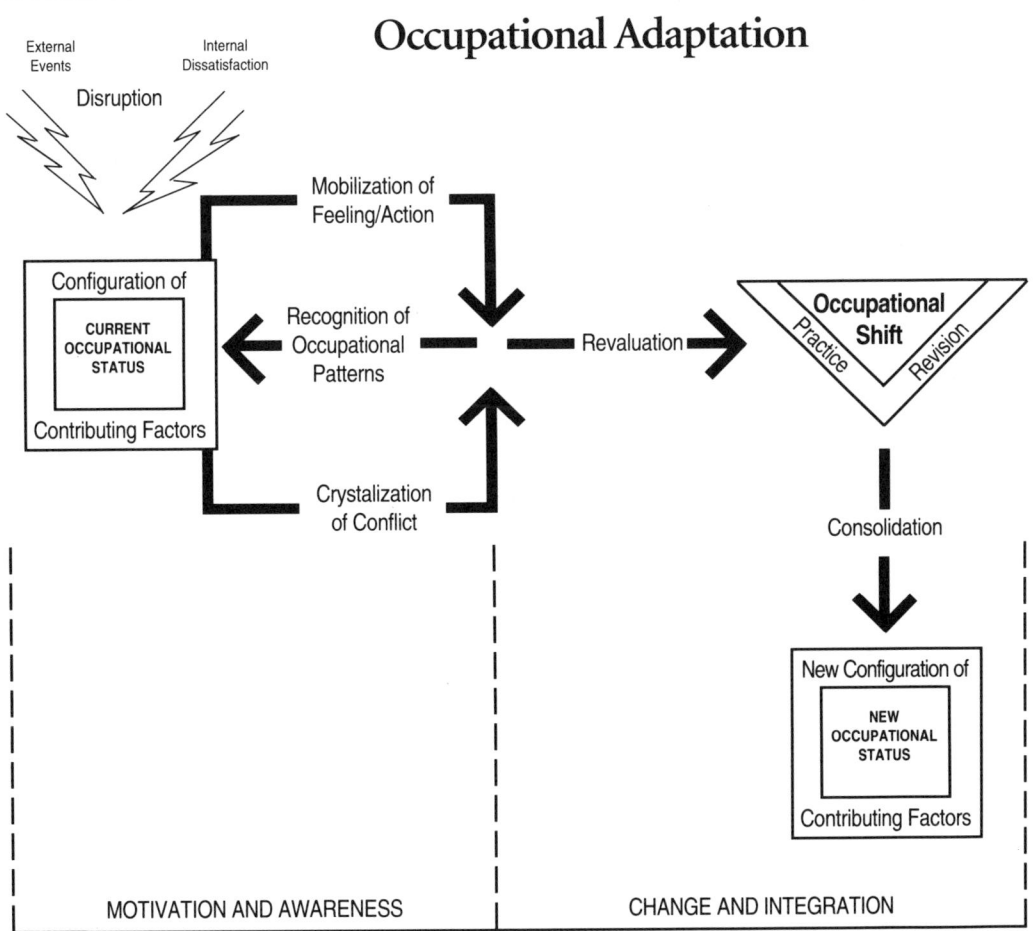

Originally appeared in Rosenfeld, M. (1992). Lifestyle education and revision for the worried well. *Work: A Journal of Prevention, Assessment, and Rehabilitation, 2*(3), 22. Adapted with permission.

the individual examines these patterns and configurations in a revaluation process. Revaluation leads to decisions and actions that constitute an occupational shift. Eventually, a consolidation of occupational functioning occurs as new behavior is revised and practiced over time.

A 48-year-old attorney traversed this process during the sessions of a *Wellness and Lifestyle Renewal* workshop. While he was successful in his career, the man felt unhappy. His wife and children complained that he was grumpy and lethargic at home. Their complaints and his dissatisfaction were disruptions in his occupational status that mobilized him to attend the workshop. Completion of a Role Checklist exercise (see p. 45) crystallized for the attorney his loss of meaning and direction, a common mid-life phenomenon. He recognized that his lethargy and grumpiness at home were reactions to his loss of active participation in formerly valued roles as a volunteer, organization member, husband, and father. The man concentrated on revaluation of his roles and leisure pursuits. After completing a collage of his future (see p. 90), he conceptualized an occupational shift. This shift included a plan to join a local church in order to increase social involvement and revitalize his spiritual life. He was also determined to volunteer for an ecological organization. The man wished to hike into wilderness areas and to improve and preserve trails. His family members were enthusiastic about joining him in this activity. The attorney felt that the changes he visualized would energize him, establish a new sense of direction, and create an avenue for positive family experiences.

The exercises that follow will lead you through the steps of the change process described above.

12.

Self-Assessment and Interpretation of Results

This chapter contains exercises that coincide with the steps of the occupational adaptation process described on page 83. Your lifestyle is viewed through a high-powered microscope at this point. Each exercise and activity will enable you to move along from recognition of lifestyle characteristics toward a resolution and a direction for change. While some people quickly establish a single focus of attention, others find several areas of concern. If the latter is true for you, you may avoid feeling overwhelmed by choosing one important area with which to begin. If you succeed in making an initial change, even a small one, you will be encouraged to tackle others thereafter. Remember, this project can last your whole life long!

Exercise

Recognition

Think carefully about your current occupational status. Rate from 1 to 5 your present degree of satisfaction regarding each element of the Model of Human Occupation listed below. Beside each item, write a phrase or sentence that explains your rating.

	very dissatisfied		average		very satisfied
Personal Causation	1	2	3	4	5
Goals and Interests	1	2	3	4	5
Spiritual Plane	1	2	3	4	5
Intellectual Plane	1	2	3	4	5
Emotional Plane	1	2	3	4	5
Physical Plane	1	2	3	4	5
Role Identifications	1	2	3	4	5
Habits/Time Use	1	2	3	4	5
Work	1	2	3	4	5
Leisure	1	2	3	4	5
Chores	1	2	3	4	5
Rest	1	2	3	4	5
Skills	1	2	3	4	5
Environments: Physical	1	2	3	4	5
Social	1	2	3	4	5
Output	1	2	3	4	5
System Trajectory	1	2	3	4	5

Now review the self-assessment you have just completed to strengthen your perspective of your current lifestyle. Be sure to notice areas of comfort and strength as well as areas of dissatisfaction. Summarize below.

My Current Lifestyle:

Exercise

Mobilization and Conflict, Part I

In this exercise, you will identify the degree to which you feel mobilized for change. In the first column next to each category, write the words *strong*, *weak*, or *none* to show how much motivation you possess to make change in that area. In the next column, write *strong*, *weak*, or *none* to indicate the amount of conflict you would face if you actually took steps to change in each area.

	Mobilization	Conflict
Personal Causation	_____	_____
Goals and Interests	_____	_____
Spiritual Plane	_____	_____
Intellectual Plane	_____	_____
Emotional Plane	_____	_____
Physical Plane	_____	_____
Role Identifications	_____	_____
Habits/Time Use	_____	_____
Work	_____	_____
Leisure	_____	_____
Chores	_____	_____
Rest	_____	_____
Skills	_____	_____
Environments: Physical	_____	_____
Social	_____	_____
Output	_____	_____
System Trajectory	_____	_____

Select the area you are most concerned with right now. Write a paragraph explaining the forces favoring and opposing change. What has shaped and maintained your pattern of behavior in this area?

My Most Important Area:

Exercise

Mobilization and Conflict, Part II (The Empty Chair)

Place two chairs facing each other. Concentrate on the most important area of change that you identified in Part I of this exercise. When you sit in one chair you will experience only the desire to change in that area. Sit in this chair. Close your eyes. Envision yourself and your life in five years. You have changed. You possess new virtues, ones that you have worked hard to adopt. Observe each of the changes you have made and notice the ripples they have caused in your life as a whole.

Now take the opposite seat. With your eyes closed, think about all of the obstacles to change you identified in Part I. See the negative consequences of change, your fears and reservations.

Now, with your eyes open, speak to the empty chair. Argue against change. Raise all of your concerns. Now change seats and perspectives. Argue in response, supporting the changes you imagined. Change seats as often as necessary.

What new understanding has this argument produced? Have you reduced the obstacles in some way?

Reactions to the Empty Chair exercise:

Exercise

Revaluation

Lerner (1979) has described the use of a magazine picture collage exercise as an assessment tool in occupational therapy practice.

Think about your identified area of concern. Now use pictures and words from magazines to create a collage that describes the way you wish your life to be two years from now. When you are finished, consider which parts of this future vision are already a part of your life, which ones feel close at hand, and which seem far from your grasp. What must you do to bring each part of this collage to life?

In addition to illustrating your vision of the future, your collage may reflect the clarity or disorganization of your wishes, ideas, and feelings; the importance of relationships in your life; and the areas of conflict inherent in your view of the future. If you are proceeding without a therapist or group leader, it may be useful to get someone you trust to look at your collage and to ask you some questions to clarify its content and meaning.

Questions

Understanding a Change

Answer the following questions to be clear about the characteristics of the change you are proposing:

What life areas and life planes are involved?

How long and strong a history does the occupational pattern you are concerned about possess?

Is your motivation to change strong? Is it internal in origin?

What obstacles stand in the way of this change?

Is first order or second order change required?

Will you change yourself, your environment, or both?

Does the proposed change involve personal causation and values, habits and roles, skills, an environmental shift, or overall system organization?

How will the change influence system trajectory and upward and downward spirals?

13.

Action Plans and Implementation

Revision and Action

It is time to commit yourself to a change. First, turn a sheet of paper sideways and draw a line from left to right across the page. This line will be the goal path along which your change will occur.

Imagine yourself as changed. Describe the way you now function in one clear sentence. Write this sentence on the far right of the line.

Beginning at the left, write the series of manageable steps you will take in proceeding toward your goal. Write these steps above the line.

Below each step and below the line, specify the tasks and activities you will undertake, the human and material resources you will require, the frequency of performance, and any other criteria for success you wish to set.

Include prospective dates for each part of your plan to be completed. Provide for acknowledgment or celebration of your efforts and accomplishments at critical points along the path of change. This validation is crucial, since change is often so gradual and uneven. Decide how you will thank the people who support your efforts to change as well.

Although your goal path may look straight and smooth, human growth actually occurs in fits and starts. You are likely to encounter conflicts, setbacks, and loss of momentum, as well as new understandings as you go. The performance of concrete tasks and activities may bring a rush of ideas, reactions, and information into your awareness. A housewife, for example, felt disappointed by her poor performance at an intermediate tennis class. After she revised her expectations and joined a beginners' class, however, she was able to thoroughly enjoy participation. Similarly, a man failed to increase the amount of leisure time he devoted to reading, even though he felt strongly motivated to do so. Joining a monthly book discussion group succeeded where other methods had failed. A chosen book and the scheduled meeting with other readers provided him with a necessary structure. As you make your efforts, don't hesitate to incorporate new methods, ideas, and objectives into you plan. Above all, stay with the process and change will occur!

Finally, be systematic, even obsessive. Keep a written log of your efforts. Use your calendar to guide you and help you keep your commitments to yourself. Integration and consolidation of new behavior patterns require a lot of practice!

Exercise

Your Marching Song

Think of your favorite popular songs. Choose one that has strong energy, one that holds positive memories and associations for you. Now write two verses of your own lyrics to go with the tune. In the first verse, describe your lifestyle dissatisfaction, your desire to change, and your doubts. In the second verse, present your plan to change, your determination, and the terrific feelings you will have when you achieve your goal.

When you need to draw extra motivation and energy from yourself, when you are discouraged, or when you want to celebrate a successful step, sing your song!

14.

References

Bacon, F. (1899). *The advancement of learning and novum organum (1605).* New York: Colonial Press.

Bandura, A. (1977). *Social learning theory.* Englewood Cliffs, NJ: Prentice-Hall.

Barris, R. (1982). Environmental interactions: An extension of the model of occupation. *American Journal of Occupational Therapy, 36,* 637-644.

Beck, A. (1976). *Cognitive therapy and the emotional disorders.* New York: International Universities Press.

Bronfenbrenner, U. (1979). *The ecology of human development.* Cambridge: Harvard University Press.

Bronowski, J. (1973) *The ascent of man.* Boston/Toronto: Little, Brown.

Brown, J. (1971). *The sacred pipe.* New York: Penguin.

Clark, P. (1979). Human development through occupation: Theoretical frameworks in contemporary occupational therapy practice, Part 1. *American Journal of Occupational Therapy, 33,* 505-514.

Cori, F. (1977). Work and creativity. In R. Simons & H. Pardes (Eds.), *Understanding human behavior in health and illness* (pp. 283-294). Baltimore, MD: Williams and Wilkins.

Crumbaugh, J. (1968). Cross validation of purpose-in-life test based on Frankl's concepts. *Journal of Individual Psychology, 24,* 74-81.

Dixon, K. (1988). Employee assistance programs: A primer for buyer and seller. *Hospital and Community Psychiatry, 39,* 623-627.

Eastman, G. (c. 1987). *Notes on the change process.* Unpublished manuscript.

Fayans, L., & Maehr, M. (1980). Attribution style, task selection, and achievement. In L. Fayans (Ed.), *Achievement motivation* (pp. 249-265). New York: Plenum.

Fidler, G., & Fidler, J. (1978). Doing and becoming: Purposeful action and self-actualization. *American Journal of Occupational Therapy, 32,* 305-310.

Frankl, V. (1963). *Man's search for meaning.* New York: Pocket Books.

Freud, S. (1930). *Civilization and its discontents.* London: Hogarth.

Hamburg, D., & Adams, J. (1967). A perspective on coping behavior. *Archives of General Psychiatry, 17,* 277-284.

Hartmann, H. (1958). *Ego psychology and the problem of adaptation.* New York: International Universities Press.

Harvey-Krefting, L. (1985). The concept of work in occupational therapy: A historical review. *American Journal of Occupational Therapy, 39,* 301-307.

Howe, M., & Briggs, A. (1982). An ecological systems model for occupational therapy. *American Journal of Occupational Therapy, 36,* 322-329.

Johnson, J. (1986). Wellness and occupational therapy. *American Journal of Occupational Therapy, 40,* 753-758.

Kielhofner, G. (1985). *A model of human occupation.* Baltimore: Williams and Wilkins.

Kielhofner, G., Barris, R., & Watts, J. (1982). Habits and habit dysfunction: A clinical perspective for psychosocial occupational therapy. *Occupational Therapy in Mental Health, 2,* 1-21.

Kielhofner, G., & Burke, J. (1980). A model of human occupation, Part 1: Conceptual framework and content. *American Journal of Occupational Therapy, 34,* 572-581.

Kohlberg, L. (1968). The child as a moral philosopher. *Psychology Today, 2,* 25-30.

Lerner, C. (1979). The magazine picture collage: Its clinical use and validity as an assessment device. *American Journal of Occupational Therapy, 33,* 500-504.

Lewin, K. (1935). *A dynamic theory of personality.* New York: McGraw-Hill.

Lidz, T. (1968). *The person.* New York: Basic Books.

Llorens, L. (1974). The effects of stress on growth and development. *American Journal of Occupational Therapy, 28,* 82-86.

Loeb, A., Beck, A., & Diggory, J. (1971). Differential effects of success and failure on depressed and non-depressed patients. *Journal of Nervous Mental Disorders, 152,* 106-114.

Lyons, B. (1984). Defining a child's zone of proximal development: Evaluation process for treatment planning. *American Journal of Occupational Therapy, 38,* 446-451.

Matsutsuyu, J. (1969). The interest checklist. *American Journal of Occupational Therapy, 23,* 323-328.

May, R. (1978). *The courage to create.* New York: Bantam Books.

Meyer, A. (1922). The philosophy of occupational therapy. *Archives of Occupational Therapy, 1,* 1-10.

Mumford, E. (1977). The special significance of work and studies on the stress of life events. In R. Simons & H. Pardes (Eds.), *Understanding human behavior in health and illness* (pp. 295-304). Baltimore, MD: Williams and Wilkins.

Oakley, F. (1984). *The role checklist.* Bethesda, MD: National Institute of Mental Health, Department of Rehabilitation Medicine.

O'Neill, N., & O'Neill, G. (1974). *Shifting gears: Finding security in a changing world.* New York: Evans.

Rider, B., Maurer, K., Peterson, C., Tyndall, D., & White, V. (1989). Occupational therapy in the promotion of health and the prevention of disability. *American Journal of Occupational Therapy, 43,* 806.

Riesman, D. (1950). *The lonely crowd.* New Haven: Yale University Press.

Rifkin, J. (1987). *Time wars.* New York: Touchstone.

Rogers, J. (1982). The spirit of independence: The evolution of a philosophy. *American Journal of Occupational Therapy, 36,* 709-715.

Rosenfeld, M. (1989). Occupational disruption and adaptation: A study of house fire victims. *American Journal of Occupational Therapy, 43,* 89-96.

Rosenfeld, M. (1990). A mid-career perspective on mental health practice. *Occupational Therapy in Mental Health, 12,* 47-61.

Rosenfeld, M. (1992). Lifestyle education and revision for the worried well. *Work: A Journal of Prevention, Assessment, and Rehabilitation, 2*(3), 21-27.

Rotter, J. (1966). Generalized expectancies for internal versus external control of reinforcement. *Psychological Monographs, 80* (Whole No. 609).

Rotter, J. (1971). External control and internal control. *Psychology Today, 5*(1), 37-42, 58-59.

Rybczynski, W. (1991). Waiting for the weekend. *The Atlantic Monthly, 268*(8), 35-52.

Schwartzberg, S. (1982). Motivation for activities of daily living: A study of selected psychiatric patients' self-reports. *Occupational Therapy in Mental Health, 2*(3), 1-26.

Scholem, G. (1965). *On the Kabalah and its symbolism.* New York: Schocken.

Seligman, M. (1975). *Helplessness: On depressions, development and death.* San Francisco: Freeman.

Sheehy, G. (1974). *Passages.* New York: Dutton.

Simon, S., Howe, L., & Kirschenbaum, H. (1972). *Values clarification.* New York: A & W Publishers.

Smith, B. (1974). Competence and adaptation. *American Journal of Occupational Therapy, 28,* 11-15.

Spinoza, B. (1970). *Ethics.* London: Dent.

Swanbrow, D. (1989). The paradox of happiness. *Psychology Today, 23,* 37-39.

Tagore, R. (1928). *Fireflies.* New York: MacMillan.

Taplin, J. (1971). Crisis theory: Critique and reformulation. *Community Mental Health Journal, 7,* 13-23.

Taylor, J. (1978). *Secret O'Life.* (Cassette PCT-34811). New York: Columbia Records.

Watenabe, S. (1968). *Activity configuration.* Regional Institute on the Evaluation Process, Final Report RSA-123-T-68. New York: American Occupational Therapy Association.

Watzlawick, P., Weakland, J., & Fisch, R. (1974). *Change: Principles of problem formation and problem resolution.* New York: Norton.

White, R. (1971). The urge toward competence. *American Journal of Occupational Therapy, 25,* 271-274.

Wolfson, H. (1950). *The philosophy of Spinoza: Unfolding the latent processes of his reasoning* (Vol. 1). New York: Schocken.